Sara Camañes-Gonzalvo
Natalia Zamora-Martínez
Verónica García-Sanz

Facial analysis in the diagnosis of orthodontic practice

Sara Camañes-Gonzalvo
Natalia Zamora-Martínez
Verónica García-Sanz

Facial analysis in the diagnosis of orthodontic practice

Development and application of three-dimensional virtual reality digital educational material.

ScienciaScripts

Imprint

Any brand names and product names mentioned in this book are subject to trademark, brand or patent protection and are trademarks or registered trademarks of their respective holders. The use of brand names, product names, common names, trade names, product descriptions etc. even without a particular marking in this work is in no way to be construed to mean that such names may be regarded as unrestricted in respect of trademark and brand protection legislation and could thus be used by anyone.

Cover image: www.ingimage.com

This book is a translation from the original published under ISBN 978-613-9-06363-5.

Publisher:
Sciencia Scripts
is a trademark of
Dodo Books Indian Ocean Ltd. and OmniScriptum S.R.L publishing group

120 High Road, East Finchley, London, N2 9ED, United Kingdom
Str. Armeneasca 28/1, office 1, Chisinau MD-2012, Republic of Moldova, Europe
Printed at: see last page
ISBN: 978-620-7-61431-8

Development and application of three-dimensional virtual reality digital educational material for facial analysis in the diagnosis of orthodontic practice.

Sara Camañes-Gonzalvo[1] , Natalia Zamora-Martínez[2] ; Verónica García-Sanz

[1]Collaborating Lecturer on the Master's Degree in Specialisation in Orthodontics. Faculty of Medicine and Dentistry. University of Valencia, Valencia, Spain.

[2]Associate Professor. Faculty of Medicine and Dentistry. University of Valencia, Valencia, Spain.

[3]Assistant Professor Doctor. Faculty of Medicine and Dentistry. University of Valencia, Valencia, Spain.

AUTHORS

Sara Camañes-Gonzalvo[1] ; Marta Delgado-García[2] ; Natalia Zamora-Martínez[3] ; Beatriz Tarazona-Álvarez[3] ; María Dolores Casaña-Ruiz[4] ; Verónica García-Sanz[5] ; Carlos Bellot-Arcís[6] ; Vanessa Paredes-Gallardo[6] .

[1]Collaborating Lecturer on the Master's Degree in Orthodontics. Faculty of Medicine and Dentistry, University of Valencia, Valencia, Spain.

[2]Master's Degree in Orthodontics. Faculty of Medicine and Dentistry, University of Valencia, Valencia, Spain.

[3]Associate Professor. Faculty of Medicine and Dentistry, Universitat de València, València, Spain.

[4]Associate Professor. Faculty of Medicine and Dentistry, University of Valencia, Valencia, Spain.

[5]Assistant Professor Doctor. Faculty of Medicine and Dentistry, University of Valencia, Valencia, Spain.

[6]Full Professor. Faculty of Medicine and Dentistry, University of Valencia, Valencia, Spain.

Table of Contents

CHAPTER 1. INTRODUCTION TO THREE-DIMENSIONAL (3D) ANALYSIS

Today's society is immersed in a digital environment that provides tools aimed at improving convenience and efficiency in everyday activities. From devices such as watches that monitor heart rate during physical activity, to home automation systems that transform the way we think about our homes, to IT tools that simplify everyday tasks. Today, digital technology has permeated all areas (Korte et al., 2020).

In the field of dentistry, a significant transformation has been observed thanks to the incorporation of digital technology. In particular, the adoption of digital software and three-dimensional (3D) analysis has revolutionised the processes of diagnosis, planning and evaluation of orthodontic and surgical treatments (Manosudprasit et al., 2017).

Historically, these diagnostic and planning procedures were carried out using photographic recordings taken from different angles and conventional two-dimensional (2D) radiographs. However, despite their simplicity and affordability, these techniques had considerable limitations. Firstly, the ability to capture projection angles of the patient relative to the camera was limited, and secondly, the quality of the images was affected by the distance between the patient and the camera. In addition, these techniques did not allow for linear measurements between reference points (Manosudprasit et al., 2017).

Anthropometry is a biological science concerned with the measurement of the human body. These measurements give information about the distribution and proportion of facial components: eyes, nose, cheeks, mouth, jaw and ears (Fleming et al., 1998.). Plastic surgeons use this data for planning plastic and reconstructive surgery. Forensic anthropologists can reconstruct an individual's appearance from a skull, identifying particular points of depth and the distances between them (Korte et al., 2020).

3D analysis has turned the world of dentistry upside down because it works at high speed, can be recorded for as long as desired and allows for a large amount of documentation to be stored in the practice.

There are all kinds of devices to record the patient's mouth in 3D, allowing us to see the bone, teeth and occlusion in detail, but when we want to carry out orthodontic treatment, the patient's physiognomy is often important in order to make certain decisions. So far, these records have been taken on the basis of photos in different positions, angles, etc., with greater or lesser quality (Korte et al., 2020).

Nowadays there is the option of recording the patient's face in detail in a simple way, with the 3D camera, in such a way that we can use it at any time, to know if that person has any asymmetry, superimpose models, CBCT, or all kinds of tests that can help us to make a diagnosis. The objective in the digital world is to be able to use the patient without depending on their presence (Manosudprasit et al., 2017).

In order to assess the reliability of such devices, it is essential to understand their accuracy and veracity, which means subjecting the software to extensive testing. It is important to note that in clinical settings, especially in orthodontics where a significant portion of the patients are children, record-taking can be challenging and accuracy can be compromised. Therefore, it is crucial to determine whether even small movements of the patient during record-taking can distort the measurements obtained (Manosudprasit et al., 2017). For example, when the patient is instructed to look forward, it is common for them to unconsciously tilt their head slightly upwards in an attempt to adopt a more upright posture.

In addition to facial assessment, it is essential to record the smile using three-dimensional devices. Nowadays, standardisation of communication between dentist and patient is essential, especially given the growing influence of the digital environment and the limited time patients have available for face-to-face consultations.

It is important to note that mobile devices tend to capture the smile in a distorted way compared to a professional camera. Lack of proper use of magnification or *zoom* can result in compression of the smile due to the focal distance of the mobile camera from the patient. In the case of self-portraits, the use of the *zoom* is often impractical, while in normal photography it is necessary to instruct the subject or have the assistance of another person to properly adjust the capture.

CHAPTER 2. ADVANTAGES OF THE 2D CAMERA OVER THE 3D CAMERA

So far, two-dimensional photometry has been the most economical method for capturing and storing facial images, however, it has several limitations. This system does not allow for linear measurements between reference points and provides only proportional data on the soft tissues of the face. On the other hand, 3D photography, with its ability to capture high-resolution colour surface recordings at relatively fast speeds, is now considered a significant advantage.

In the early years of 2D facial photogrammetry, Farkas et al. (1980) conducted a comparative study of facial distances, angles and inclinations. The results indicated that 41.9% of the measurements studied were considered reliable in photography, with facial inclinations being the most important. On the other hand, Han et al. (2010) conducted similar research that contradicted these findings by demonstrating a greater similarity in linear measurements.

Astudillo-Loyola et al., (2018) analysed the influence of the camera on indirect 2D and direct measurements. The authors determined an average difference of 0.9 mm with some of the measurements showing up to 2.2 mm difference using a 50 mm lens.

However, with a 100 mm lens, this average difference was reduced to between 0 mm and 1.3 mm, with an average of 0.5 mm.

The usefulness of 2D models is restricted, as their relevance is limited to the planning and prediction of the facial profile. In everyday life, the observation of patients is not limited to the profile alone, but involves a variety of perspectives. This limitation is particularly evident in the complexity of some proposed registration methods, which have serious shortcomings in terms of applicability and accuracy (Naudi et al., 2013). It is essential to recognise these limitations and explore alternative approaches that more comprehensively address the complexity of facial anatomy and clinical needs.

CHAPTER 3. 3D CAMERA UTILITIES

Continuing technological advances in 3D imaging techniques have generated increasing interest in orthognathic surgery planning, as they are considered ideal methods for facial representation (Naudi et al., 2013). Interest in the *Surgery First Approach* (SFA) approach has also increased significantly. Simulation using 3D imaging allows practitioners to plan treatment and diagnosis with greater precision and accuracy. This technique enables early aesthetic improvements in the face, an increase in the speed of movement in subsequent orthodontic treatment due to the phenomenon of regional acceleration, as well as improved stability and patient satisfaction (Camini et al., 2021).

Soft tissue reconstruction is particularly useful for simulating the behaviour of hard tissues in the face, measuring soft tissue thicknesses in various regions and predicting the approximate response to hard tissue relocations. Techniques such as stereophotogrammetry, laser scanning and structured light are now used to accurately and non-invasively capture soft tissue skin in the facial region, and the data obtained from this capture can be fully integrated with cone beam computed tomography (CBCT) data (Palomo et al., 2021).

The 3D camera is a highly versatile device that, in addition to its usefulness in orthognathic surgery, allows a comprehensive view of the patient to be obtained in other fields. Heike et al. (2010) emphasised that it is up to the reader and the user to determine the application of these techniques, whether for research purposes or to address a specific clinical question.

CHAPTER 4. 3D CAMERA TYPES

1. <u>TYPES OF 3D CAMERAS</u>

1.1. CBCT

1.1.1. KAVO 3D EXAM CBCT SCANNER

3D camera that allows the head to be scanned by CBCT, the scan is performed with the patient's head parallel to the Frankfurt plane, with a *voxel* size of 0.3 mm and a field of view of 17 mm. The DICOM files are transmitted to the software so that the image can be superimposed on the CBCT (Fourie et al., 2011).

1.2. LASER SCANNER

Düppe et al., (2018) presented this type of camera as a highly promising tool. However, this method had some limitations. One of the challenges is to keep the subject still for at least 17 seconds, which in some cases requires sedation of certain patients, making this process an invasive imaging source.

Ayoub et al., (2007) and Khambay et al., (2008) agreed that these cameras have certain limitations; the capture speed is slower compared to other methods, which may result in image distortions due to subject movement or changes in facial expression. In addition, they noted that the images of the skin surface lack photographic realism and the characteristic texture of the skin.

1.2.1. MINOLTA VIVID 900 (OSAKA, JAPAN)

The laser scanner, equipped with a head positioning bracket, operates by scanning frontally, 45° to the right and 45° to the left of the patient. These images are further processed and stored on an external hard drive (Fourie, et al., 2011).

1.3. 3D STEREO PHOTOGRAMMETRY

The three-dimensional image is generated by using a set of cameras and a flash unit positioned at specific locations. When all units are activated simultaneously, a 3D image is automatically generated. According to Düppe et al. (2018), this method has great potential for assessing the anatomical dimensions and proportions of a subject. A notable advantage is the ability to capture virtually instantaneous images and its ease of integration into medical practice.

The designated space should be sufficient to accommodate the entire system and the subject without obstruction during the capture process. Factors such as the availability of an adequate power supply, internet access and network connection points, as well as the flow of pedestrian traffic in the area, should be considered. It is desirable for the operator to be able to view the computer screen during the capture process. A permanent installation offers advantages such as reduced equipment degradation, greater consistency in data collection, improved quality and significant time savings.

It is important to take into account the difficulty these systems face in accurately capturing hair and avoiding artefacts that may be caused by objects or subject accessories. Therefore, the patient shall be instructed to take the necessary measures to avoid substantial loss of surface data on the head and face.

During image capture, it is essential that the subject maintains a neutral facial expression. In some cases, the use of an object may help to fix the subject's gaze in the optimal direction.

Many such systems operate using a single frontal 3D capture of the face, resulting in reliable data covering a viewing angle of 160 to 180 degrees. However, this modality can be limited in terms of the quality of the frontal capture. Some modular systems offer the possibility to extend the coverage up to 360 degrees, which leads to increased costs and space requirements.

Adequate lighting is another crucial requirement for these photography systems. While lighting conditions in office environments are generally acceptable, excessively high or low levels of ambient light can saturate the camera sensors. The use of internal or external *flash* mechanisms can mitigate this problem, but the layout of the system needs to be considered to avoid interference with external light (Heike et al., 2010).

Heike et al., (2010) emphasised that certain anatomical regions, such as the subnasal and submental area, can be difficult to capture, which can result in loss of data and artefacts in the images. To accurately assess the asymmetry or morphology of the nostrils, it is essential that the subject slightly tilts the head during image capture.

Fourie et al. (2011) described the inherent advantages of this type of camera, emphasising its ability to take snapshots in an exceptionally short time of 1.5 milliseconds, which helps to minimise the risk of movement during image capture. In addition, the associated software offers tools that allow image manipulation, thus facilitating the identification of reference points and the precise calculation of measurements and volumes.

1.3.1. Di3D (DIMENSIONAL IMAGING)

Capable of generating high-resolution, full-colour, three-dimensional models with a 180-degree, ear-to-ear view within 180 seconds, this system consists of two interconnected camera stations. Each station includes a pair of high-resolution digital cameras and two white light *flash units*, placed adjacent to the respective stations. Before each use, the system has to be calibrated by an automated procedure. This system has been used in several studies (Khambay et al., 2008; Fourie et al., 2011).

Fourie et al., (2008) highlighted the ability to resolve details of linear densities close to 0.1 mm per pixel in human faces. On the other hand, Khambay et al., (2008), in their study, validated this claim with a technical accuracy within the range of 0.2 mm, which is considered clinically acceptable.

1.3.2. 3dMDDface System (3dMD, Atlanta)

This system is composed of four geometric cameras and two texture cameras, arranged in a triangular shape with three cameras on each side. During each image capture, the camera views are synchronised and software algorithms merge the different overlapping images to generate a single three-dimensional image. This resulting image can be visualised, manipulated and analysed on a computer.

Each image is composed of high-resolution 3D surface geometry, including x, y, and z coordinates, as well as colour and texture information. This system has been used in several studies (Weinberg et al., 2006; Wong et al., 2008).

1.3.3. Genex

This system emits structured light onto the surface of an object to generate and capture three-dimensional information (Weingberg et al., 2006).

1.3.4. Morpheus 3D

The camera operates similarly to the Genex, with a capture time of 0.8 seconds and an accuracy of less than 0.1 mm according to the manufacturer. Three photographs of the subject are required: one front and two side shots, each taken at a 45-degree angle.

These images are combined to form a unified three-dimensional representation. Kim et al. (2015) performed measurements using the line length tool in the Morpheus 3D camera's own software, taking direct measurements between two points. The discrepancy between the two methods was less than 1 mm.

CHAPTER 5. 3D CAMERA OPERATION

For an accurate analysis of the subject, it is important to ensure correct positioning and reference when capturing the image. In the literature, the 3D image processing process is based on 2D cephalometric record capture and planning, using the Frankfurt plane as a reference point and orientation.

This plane is consistently selected because the facebow transfer also mirrors the axioorbital plane, which facilitates alignment of the models in the joint, ensuring internal consistency.

In the three-dimensional context, it is not appropriate to rely solely on a line connecting the orbital and porion points, as these elements are duplicated. It is therefore essential to establish planes rather than lines. For this purpose, several planes can be used, including the Frankfurt plane, the mid-sagittal plane and the transporionic plane.

This orientation approach optimally approximates the natural position of the head, thus ensuring the accuracy and reliability of the analysis performed.

Palomo et al., (2021), in their study, mention several computer programmes that allow the user to plot orientation landmarks on the craniofacial skeleton and teeth, using data obtained from the clinical physical analysis to reproduce the natural head position (NCP). Head orientation can also be adjusted with manual orientation tools, rotation, roll and pitch controls. The accuracy of the final orientation can be confirmed by comparisons with extraoral photographs taken using the true vertical line.

To help the subject adopt their PNC, there are laser light indicators, gyroscopic positioners placed in the mouth and linked to electronic referencing devices, as well as the placement of markers. According to Caminiti (2021), the PNC can vary by up to 8°, and this discrepancy can be responsible for a 15% difference in maxillary projection between planned and actual results.

Historically, several studies have emphasised that the natural position of the head should be considered as the initial position for photography, in contrast to other parameters based on intracranial references such as the Frankfurt plane, which show a remarkable variability (Cooke et al., 1990; Lundstöm et al., 1995; Peng et al., 1999; Madsen et al., 2008).

1. PROTOCOL FOR REVIEWING A PROPER 3D FACIAL CAPTURE (Heike et al., 2010).

- Is the subject's facial expression neutral?

- Is there evidence of unwanted movement in the catch?

- Are there signs of interference (e.g. scalp hair) or artefacts affecting image quality?

- Is the picture quality satisfactory?

- Is there adequate surface coverage of the facial regions targeted by the clinical or research study?

2. SUMMARY OF RECOMMENDATIONS FOR OPTIMISING IMAGE ACQUISITION (Heike et al., 2010).

1) Select a large space for unobstructed image flow and sufficient ambient lighting.

2) Select seats that are appropriate for your population and that facilitate quick positioning. When working with children, choose seating options that allow for maximum flexibility and safety.

3) Before capturing the image, reposition any scalp hair that obscures the relevant anatomical surface and remove all reflective objects.

4) Work with the subject to achieve a "neutral" facial expression. If images are taken before and after the operation, ask the subject to repeat their expression.

5) To maximise coverage of the facial surface, position the patient's head so that priority areas are visible to the system's cameras or consider additional captures from alternative views.

6) Consider batch image processing when many images have to be taken in a limited time.

CHAPTER 6. DESIGN AND IMPLEMENTATION OF 3D ANALYSIS AS A TEACHING MATERIAL IN DENTISTRY - INTRODUCTION AND OBJECTIVES

1. INTRODUCTION

In the field of dentistry, the introduction of digital software and three-dimensional (3D) dental and facial analysis has radically transformed the approach to dental diagnosis and treatment planning (Genaro et al., 2021). This evolution has enabled a more complete and detailed view of the oral and facial anatomy, which is essential for accurate and efficient clinical practice.

Traditionally, these diagnostic and planning processes were based on two-dimensional (2D) photographic and radiographic recordings, which, despite their utility and economy, had significant limitations. These limitations included the difficulty in adequately visualising lateral areas of the face and the inability to make linear measurements between key anatomical points. These limitations not only affected professional practice, but also had a direct impact on the academic training of dental students, hindering their learning process and understanding of oral and facial anatomy (De Juan et al., 2013).

In the context of the 21st century, society is immersed in a digital environment that has transformed the way we perform both our personal and professional tasks (Genaro et al., 2021). In this sense, it is essential to assess the feasibility of incorporating 3D technology into preclinical dental practices. This represents a significant advance that could substantially improve the training of future dentists by providing them with advanced tools for more accurate diagnosis and more effective treatment planning (Paredes-Gallardo et al., 2014).

In addition, the integration of 3D technology into the dental curriculum could bring standards of excellence in dental care even closer, thereby improving clinical outcomes and patient experience.

The implementation of multimedia teaching materials and 3D virtual reality models in the university educational environment represents a significant innovation that offers numerous benefits for student learning. These technological tools not only serve as complementary resources to reinforce theoretical concepts taught in the classroom, but also foster autonomous learning by providing students with the opportunity to explore and practice interactively (Paredes-Gallardo et al., 2014; Gerano et al., 2021).

Specifically, digitisation of craniometric point measurements and linear measurements of facial thirds offers accuracy in the assessment of patient proportionality. By allowing three-dimensional visualisation of the data, these digital tools provide a spatial perspective that is not possible with traditional 2D methods. This enhanced ability to analyse and understand facial anatomy facilitates both the learning process and the diagnostic ability of students, better preparing them for their future professional practice (Tarazona-Alvarez et al., 2015).

2. OBJECTIVES OF THE TEACHING INNOVATION PROJECT

2.1. MAIN OBJECTIVES

The fundamental purpose of this project is to develop, implement and refine virtual reality resources aimed at improving the quality of learning for dental students in order to prepare them for their future professional practice. To achieve this goal, the most advanced and innovative resources currently available in the field of educational technology will be used.

One of the main objectives of this project is to integrate 3D diagnostic tools, such as three-dimensional photographs, into the curriculum of the Degree in Dentistry at the University of Valencia. This early integration into the academic training will allow students to become familiar with these technologies and develop advanced skills in dental diagnosis and treatment. Furthermore, by exposing students to these tools from early stages of their training, the aim is to better prepare them to face the challenges and demands of professional practice in an increasingly digitised and technologically advanced healthcare environment.

2.2. SPECIFIC OBJECTIVES

In addition to the general objectives mentioned above, this study set out to achieve a number of specific objectives that would contribute to a deeper and more detailed understanding of the effectiveness and perceptions of the teaching methodologies employed. These specific objectives are detailed below:

1. To compare the effectiveness of two teaching methodologies: a traditional one, in which students must identify a series of craniometric points on 2D front and profile photographs and perform a facial analysis, and an innovative one, which uses a 3D virtual reality model where students must locate the craniometric points and perform a facial analysis.

2. To assess the students' opinion of the two methodologies (traditional and virtual reality) through an anonymous survey

with closed questions, administered through virtual learning platforms.

3. To obtain teachers' opinions on the two methodologies by means of an anonymous survey including closed questions, with the aim of understanding their perception of the effectiveness and usefulness of each pedagogical approach.

4. Carry out a comparative analysis of the two methodologies used, evaluating their effectiveness and usefulness as learning tools. This analysis will allow us to identify the strengths and weaknesses of each approach and produce improvements in the design and implementation of educational strategies in the dental field.

CHAPTER 7. DESIGN AND IMPLEMENTATION OF 3D ANALYSIS AS A TEACHING MATERIAL IN DENTISTRY - METHODOLOGY

3. <u>METHODOLOGY</u>

3.1. Tools for facial analysis

For the execution of the facial analysis exercise using virtual reality, a three-dimensional image is required, which is acquired using a dedicated camera such as the Bellus 3D Face Camera Pro® , which has the ability to capture a complete and detailed representation of the facial structure (Figure 1). This approach, as opposed to conventional two-dimensional photographs, provides a more accurate and detailed visualisation of facial features, which is essential for a comprehensive analysis.

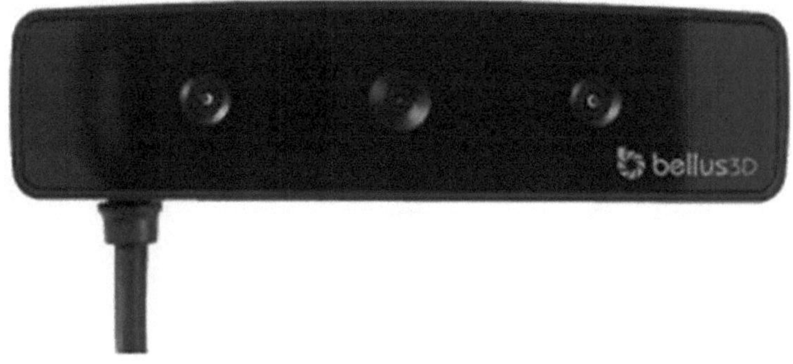

Figure 1. Camera used to perform the 3D facial analysis. Bellus 3D Face Camera Pro® .

Three-dimensional image processing and analysis is usually performed through specialised software, such as Dolphin Imaging 11.95 Premium® or Invivo Dental 6.0® (Anatomage, San Jose, CA) (Figure 2). These platforms offer advanced tools that allow accurate measurements and detailed analysis of various facial structures, providing a solid basis for diagnosis and treatment planning in dentistry.

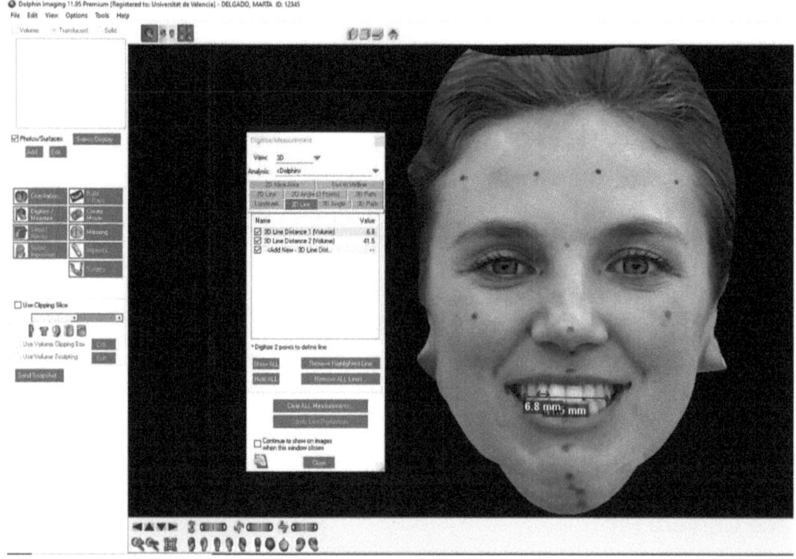

Figure 2. Performing measurements for facial analysis using Dolphin Imaging 11.95 Premium software® .

In addition to these options, there are also publicly available 3D measurement tools that can be used for educational and clinical purposes. This variety of resources provides students with the opportunity to familiarise themselves with different facial analysis tools and techniques, thus enriching their learning experience and preparing them to face the challenges of clinical practice with confidence and competence.

3.2. Didactic procedure

The educational process is structured as follows:

1. <u>DESCRIPTION OF THE ANTHROPOMETRIC POINTS AND
LINEAR MEASUREMENTS USED.</u>

For the study, 24 craniometric points and 16 linear measurements were used. These points and linear measurements are based on a study with a similar design which in turn is based on the points described by Farkas et al (1980).

1.1. ANTHROPOMETRIC POINTS

The 24 craniometric points used were as follows:

- N: Nasion - Point on the midline of the intersection of the root of the nose and the frontonasal suture.
- Al: Right and left wing (right and left) - Most lateral point of the outline of the wing of the nose.
- Pn: Pronasal - Most protruding point of the tip of the nose identified in lateral view with the head in the resting position.
- Sn: Subnasal - Midpoint of the angle of the base of the columella where the lower edge of the nasal septum and the surface of the upper lip meet.
- Ls: Upper lip - Midpoint of the vermilion line of the upper lip.

- Stm: Stomion - Imaginary point where the vertical facial midline and the labial fissure intersect when the lips are in contact without forcing.

- Ch: Chelion (right and left) - Most lateral point of the vermilion border at the corner of the patient's mouth.

- B': Sublabial - Lower edge of lower lip or upper edge of chin.

- Pog': Pogonion - Most anterior point at the midpoint of the chin.

- Tra: Tragion (right and left) - Point at the upper margin of the tragus of the ear.

- En: Endocanthion (right and left) - Inner corner of the eye.

- Ex: Exocanthion (right and left) - Outermost point of the corner of the eye.

- Ck: Cheek (right and left) - Intersection point of the lines connecting Al-Tra and Ex-Ch.

- La1, La2, La3 and La4: - Points located 5 mm above the right and left Ex and right and left En.

1.2. LINEAR MEASUREMENTS

The 16 linear measurements used were as follows (Figure 3):

- Ex - Ex: (distance from right Exocanthion to left Exocanthion).

- In - In: (distance from right Endocanthion to left Endocanthion).

- Al - Al: (distance from right wing to left wing).

- Ch - Ch: (distance from right Chelion to left Chelion).

- Tra - Ck: (distance from Tragion to Cheek right and left).

- N - Pn: (distance from Nasion to Pronasal).

- Pn - Sn: (distance from Pronasal to Subnasal).

- Sn - Ls: (distance from Subnasal to Upper lip).

- Sn - Stm: (distance from Subnasal to Stomion).

- Stm - Pog': (distance from Stomion to Pogonion).

- Stm - B: (distance from Pogonion to Sublabial).

- La1 - La2: (distance from La1 to La2).

- La3 - La4: (distance from La3 to La4).

- Al - Ch: (distance from Alar to Chelion right and left).

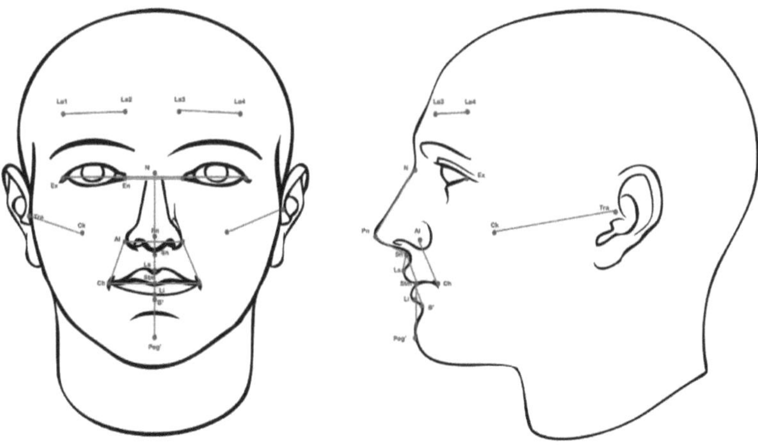

Figure 3. Linear measurements

The naming of the points has been based on Greek or Latin anatomical terminology, and lower case abbreviations have been used to distinguish them from cephalometric hard tissue points. Correct selection and identification of these anatomical points, regardless of the measurement or scanning technique used, is essential for direct and indirect measurements in 2D and 3D imaging.

2. ASSESSMENT OF FACIAL PROPORTIONS

After the correct location of the above-mentioned points, the facial proportions are assessed. In this facial analysis, the focus is on the study of the vertical proportions of the face. For this purpose, the face is divided into three thirds: upper, middle and lower. The upper third extends from the Trichion point to the Glabella point; the middle third extends from the Glabella point to the Subnasal point; and finally, the lower third extends from the Subnasal point to the Gnation point.

3. LOCATING THE POINTS AND TAKING THE FACIAL MEASUREMENTS ON THE 2D PHOTO

In order to carry out the location of the facial points on the 2D photograph, the students are required to have two printed images, which are included in the "Orthodontic Practice Guide I". In the practical process, students are required to meticulously identify each of the points on both images, both in frontal and lateral view, using a fine-tipped pencil. Also, measurements of facial proportions are made manually, using a millimetre ruler to ensure the accuracy of the data obtained.

4. LOCATING POINTS AND PERFORMING FACIAL MEASUREMENTS ON 3D VIRTUAL REALITY MODELS

In this context, facial analysis measurements are carried out directly in freely accessible software. On this platform, students have the ability to manipulate the three-dimensional image by rotating, panning and zooming as needed. This functionality allows them to adjust the visualisation for precise localisation of anatomical points, which is done individually for each student.

In contrast, in the case of 3D photography, it is not necessary to capture two separate records. A single image is sufficient to locate all points corresponding to the orbital, nasal, buccal and auricular regions. This is because the three-dimensional image encompasses all areas of facial interest, thus simplifying the process of locating anatomical points.

CHAPTER 8. DESIGN AND IMPLEMENTATION OF 3D ANALYSIS AS A TEACHING MATERIAL IN DENTISTRY - RESULTS

This work concluded with the implementation of an innovative methodology aimed at improving the facial analysis process in orthodontic patients through the use of three-dimensional tools. This initiative was designed with the purpose of equipping dental students, particularly those enrolled in the subject Orthodontics I, with skills and abilities adapted to the current demands of the field of dentistry.

Prior to the pre-clinical facial analysis exercises, two specially designed explanatory videos were produced and presented and discussed with the students. Afterwards, a detailed explanation of the new methodology was given by the lecturer in charge of the practical exercises. Subsequently, the students proceeded to practice using both methodologies: firstly, carrying out the traditional two-dimensional analysis using conventional photographs, and then using the new 3D tools.

To assess participant satisfaction, structured surveys were administered as checklists, with respondents indicating their level of agreement on a scale of 0 to 3, where 0 represents "never", 1 "sometimes", 2 "often" and 3 "always" (see Tables 1 and 2). This approach allowed all the specific objectives to be met.

Table 1. Survey to be completed by students. Comparison of 2D and 3D tools. Effectiveness and usefulness.

		0	1	2	3
EVALUATION TEMPLATE AUMNADO					
1	Access to the teaching videos through the Virtual Classroom space is simple.				
2	Downloading this resource from the Virtual Classroom is easy and accessible to all members of the subject.				
3	I find the use of videos explaining the new methodology interesting from an educational point of view.				
4	Performing facial analysis with 3D tools has increased my diagnostic knowledge.				
5	Thanks to the comparison between methodologies, I have been able to learn about the differences between them.				
6	The content of the internships is adequate and well structured.				
7	The images included help to better understand the theoretical concepts.				
8	I found it easy to carry out the practical exercises using 3D tools.				
9	I would advise change through the new 3D tools for facial diagnosis.				
10	I think I could apply the knowledge I have acquired to my profession.				

Table 2. Survey to be completed by teachers. Effectiveness and usefulness.

		0	1	2	3
TEACHER EVALUATION TEMPLATE					
1	The development of teaching videos is a simple process.				
2	Uploading the videos to the Virtual Classroom is interesting from a didactic point of view.				
3	The incorporation of 3D tools has been a time-consuming effort.				
4	I consider that the implementation of these tools has been very useful for the development of new skills by the students.				
5	Once implemented, I would use this methodology again for the next school year.				

The data collected through the surveys reflected a high level of satisfaction on the part of the participants in all the aspects evaluated, showing positive results in each of the sections analysed, as illustrated in detail in Figures 4 and 5.

The findings revealed a favourable reception of the new methodology implemented, highlighting the perceived efficacy of the orthodontic facial analysis process using three-dimensional tools.

There was also a clear preference for this innovative approach compared to the traditional two-dimensional method, suggesting a recognition by students of the benefits inherent in the use of advanced technologies in the field of dentistry.

These results validate the effectiveness of the implemented pedagogical strategy and support its integration into the dental degree curriculum as an effective and well-received training tool for students.

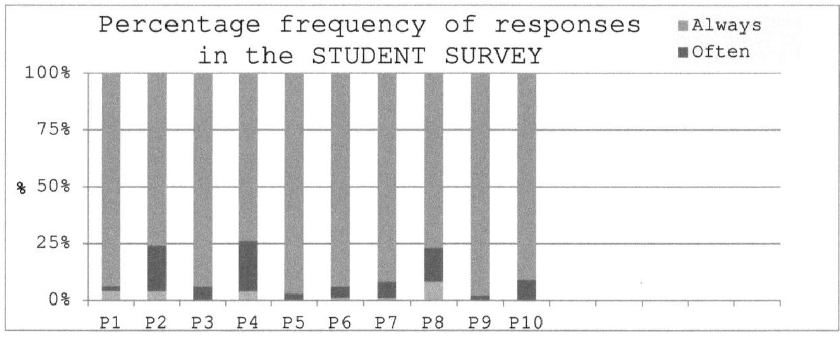

Figure 4. Results of the surveys filled in by students

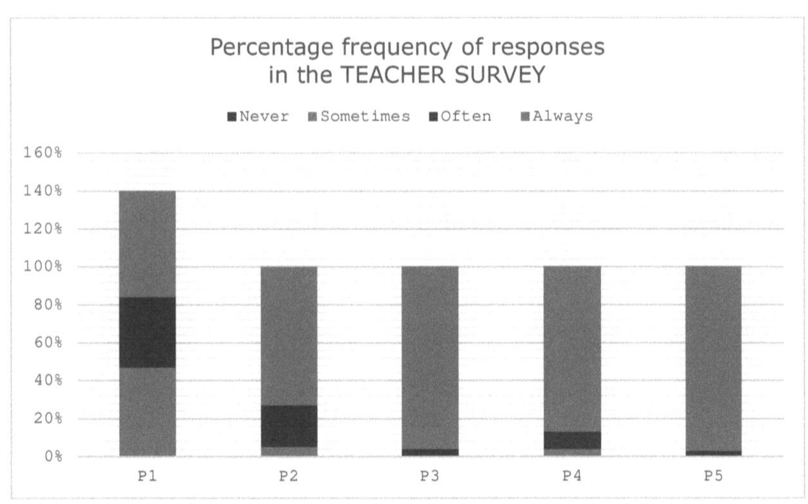

Figure 5. Results of the surveys completed by teachers

CHAPTER 9. DESIGN AND IMPLEMENTATION OF 3D ANALYSIS AS A TEACHING MATERIAL IN DENTISTRY - CONCLUSIONS AND IMPACT

The positive impact generated by the implementation of three-dimensional tools for 3D facial analysis during the practical sessions of the subject Orthodontics I was reflected in the academic performance of the students, showing notable improvements in the results of the exams and in the marks obtained in the practical sessions. These tools not only served as didactic support during the practical sessions, but also facilitated the assimilation of the theoretical concepts related to the subject, thus contributing to a deeper and more complete understanding of the contents.

Access to these new three-dimensional facial analysis tools represented a significant advance in the development and study of the subject of Orthodontics I, providing students with an innovative and highly efficient way of learning. The incorporation of multimedia technologies in the teaching-learning process not only speeded up the acquisition of knowledge, but also promoted the standardisation and protocolisation of practices, thus guaranteeing comprehensive, quality training for the students.

It is important to highlight that this project had a significant impact on a considerable number of students, given that the Orthodontics I subject usually has an annual enrolment of between 70 and 80 students. The implementation of these tools represented an important step towards the modernisation and continuous improvement of teaching in the dental field, providing students with an enriching learning experience adapted to the demands of the digital era.

BIBLIOGRAPHICAL REFERENCES

1. Korte, M. (2020) The impact of the digital revolution on human brain and behavior: where do we stand? Dialogues Clinical Neurosciences, 22(2), 101-111.

2. Manosudprasit, A., Haghi, A., Veerasathpurush Allareddy, V., Masoud, M. I. (2017). Diagnosis and treatment planning of orthodontic patients with 3-dimensional dentofacial records. American Journal of Orthodontics and Dentofacial Orthopedics,Volume 151, Issue 6.

3. Fleming, B., & Dobbs, D. (1998). Animating facial features and expressions. Charles River Media, Inc.

4. Farkas, L. G., Bryson, W., & Klotz, J. (1980). Is photogrammetry of the face reliable? Plastic and Reconstructive surgery, 66(3), 346-355.

5. Han, K., Kwon, H. J., Choi, T. H., Kim, J. H., & Son, D. (2010). Comparison of anthropometry with photogrammetry based on a standardized clinical photographic technique using a cephalostat and chair. Journal of Cranio-Maxillofacial Surgery, 38(2), 96-107.

6. Astudillo-Loyola, M. P., Dehghan-Manshadi-Kemm, S., Vergara-Nuñez, C., & Peñafiel-Ekdhal, C. (2018). Are photographs reliable for facial analysis in orthodontics? Clinical journal of periodontology, implantology and oral rehabilitation, 11(1), 13-15.

7. Naudi, K. B., Benramadan, R., Brocklebank, L., Ju, X., Khambay, B., & Ayoub, A. (2013). The virtual human face: superimposing the simultaneously captured 3D photorealistic skin surface of the face on the untextured skin image of the

CBCT scan. International journal of oral and maxillofacial surgery, 42(3), 393-400.

8. Caminiti, M., & Lou, T. (2021). 3D Planning for Complex Cases in Orthognathic Surgery. In 3D Diagnosis and Treatment Planning in Orthodontics (pp. 283-297). Springer, Cham.

9. Caminiti, M. (2021). Digital Planning in Orthognathic Surgery. In 3D Diagnosis and Treatment Planning in Orthodontics (pp. 267-282). Springer, Cham.

10. Palomo, J. M., El, H., Stefanovic, N., Eliliwi, M., Elshebiny, T., & Pugliese, F. (2021). 3D Cephalometry. In 3D Diagnosis and Treatment Planning in Orthodontics (pp. 93-127). Springer, Cham.

11. Heike, C. L., Upson, K., Stuhaug, E., & Weinberg, S. M. (2010). 3D digital stereophotogrammetry: a practical guide to facial image acquisition. Head & face medicine, 6(1), 1-11.

12. Fourie, Z., Damstra, J., Gerrits, P. O., & Ren, Y. (2011). Evaluation of anthropometric accuracy and reliability using different three-dimensional scanning systems. Forensic science international, 207(1-3), 127-134.

13. Düppe, K., Becker, M., & Schönmeyr, B. (2018). Evaluation of facial anthropometry using three-dimensional photogrammetry and direct measuring techniques. Journal of Craniofacial Surgery, 29(5), 1245-1251.

14. Ayoub, A. F., Xiao, Y., Khambay, B., Siebert, J. P., & Hadley, D. (2007). Towards building a photo-realistic virtual human face for craniomaxillofacial diagnosis and treatment planning. International journal of oral and maxillofacial surgery, 36(5), 423-428.

15.   Khambay, B., Nairn, N., Bell, A., Miller, J., Bowman, A., & Ayoub, A. F. (2008). Validation and reproducibility of a high-resolution three-dimensional facial imaging system. British Journal of Oral and Maxillofacial Surgery, 46(1), 27-32.

16.   Weinberg, S. M., Naidoo, S., Govier, D. P., Martin, R. A., Kane, A. A., & Marazita, M. L. (2006). Anthropometric precision and accuracy of digital three-dimensional photogrammetry: comparing the Genex and 3dMD imaging systems with one another and with direct anthropometry. Journal of Craniofacial Surgery, 17(3), 477-483.

17.   Wong, J. Y., Oh, A. K., Ohta, E., Hunt, A. T., Rogers, G. F., Mulliken, J. B., & Deutsch, C. K. (2008). Validity and reliability of craniofacial anthropometric measurement of 3D digital photogrammetric images. The Cleft Palate-Craniofacial Journal, 45(3), 232-239.

18.   Kim, S. H., Jung, W. Y., Seo, Y. J., Kim, K. A., Park, K. H., & Park, Y. G. (2015). Accuracy and precision of integumental linear dimensions in a three-dimensional facial imaging system. The korean journal of orthodontics, 45(3), 105-112.

19.   Cooke, M. S., & Orth, D. (1990). Five-year reproducibility of natural head posture: a longitudinal study. American Journal of Orthodontics and Dentofacial Orthopedics, 97(6), 489-494.

20.   Lundström, A., Lundström, F., Lebret, L. M. L., & Moorrees, C. F. A. (1995). Natural head position and natural head orientation: basic considerations in cephalometric analysis and research. European Journal of Orthodontics, 17(2), 111-120.

21.   Peng, L., & Cooke, M. S. (1999). Fifteen-year reproducibility of natural head posture: a longitudinal study.

American Journal of Orthodontics and Dentofacial Orthopedics, 116(1), 82-85.

22.   Madsen, D. P., Sampson, W. J., & Townsend, G. C. (2008). Craniofacial reference plane variation and natural head position. The European Journal of Orthodontics, 30(5), 532-540.

23.   Genaro, Luis Eduardo, & Capote, Ticiana Sidorenko de Oliveira (2021). Use of virtual reality in dentistry: literature review. Odovtos International Journal of Dental Sciences, 23(2), 33-38.

24.   De Juan, J., Pérez-Cañaveras, R.M., Girela, J.L., Vizcaya, M.F., Segovia, Y., Romero, A., Martínez, A. (2013). Importance of the use of didactic videos in face-to-face teaching of Biology subjects. In XI Jornadas de redes de investigación en docencia universitaria (pp. 610-23).

25.   Paredes Gallardo, V., Tarazona Álvarez, B., Zamora Martínez, N., Bellot Arcís, C. (2014). Multimedia videos as a learning tool in the dentist-patient relationship in the Degree in Dentistry. In Nuevas formulaciones de los contenidos docentes. McGraw-Hill, Spain, ISBN 978- 84-481-9739-1.

26.   Tarazona Álvarez, B., Paredes Gallardo, V., Zamora Martínez, N., Bellot Arcís, C. (2015) Animations in three dimensions as a tool for teaching innovation in the Degree in Dentistry. Evaluation of the Quality of Research and Higher Education: book of abstracts XI FECIES / coord. by María Teresa Ramiro Sánchez, Tamara Ramiro Sánchez, ISBN 978-84-697-1002-9, pp. 607-607.

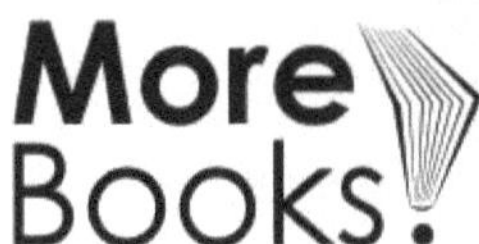

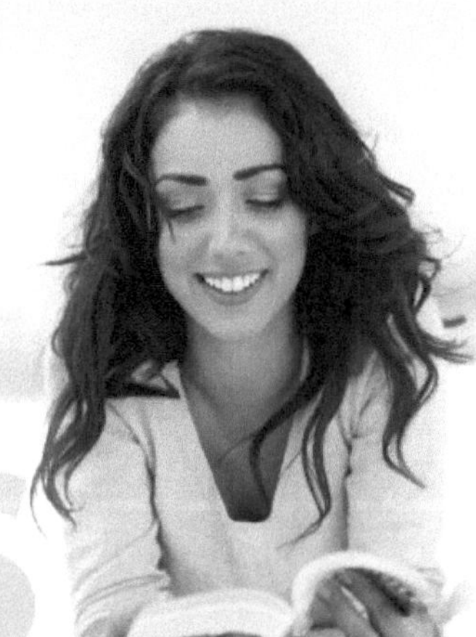

I want morebooks!

Buy your books fast and straightforward online - at one of world's fastest growing online book stores! Environmentally sound due to Print-on-Demand technologies.

Buy your books online at
www.morebooks.shop

Kaufen Sie Ihre Bücher schnell und unkompliziert online – auf einer der am schnellsten wachsenden Buchhandelsplattformen weltweit! Dank Print-On-Demand umwelt- und ressourcenschonend produzi ert.

Bücher schneller online kaufen
www.morebooks.shop

info@omniscriptum.com
www.omniscriptum.com

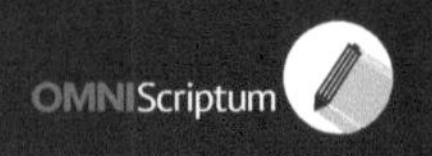

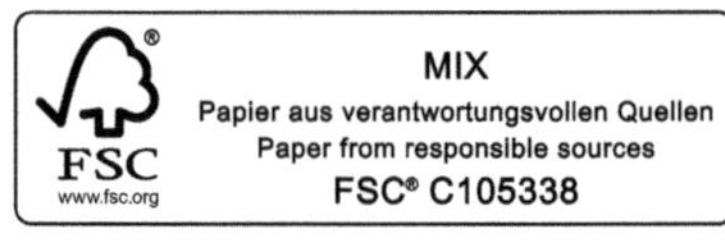

Printed by Books on Demand GmbH, Norderstedt / Germany